JUICING FOR CANCER RECIPES BOOK

"Fueling Your Fight: Delicious Juices to Support Cancer Treatment and Recovery"

Michael J. Green

TABLE OF CONTENT

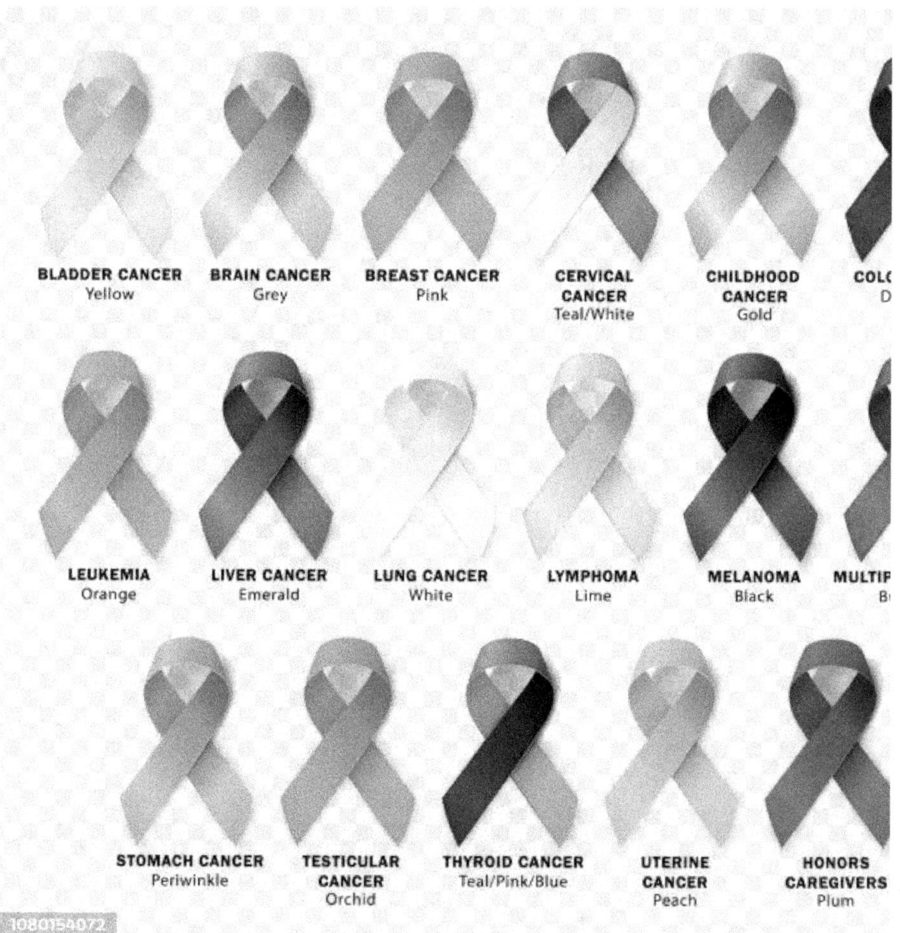

BLADDER CANCER
Yellow
BRAIN CANCER
Grey
BREAST CANCER
Pink
CERVICAL CANCER
Teal/White
CHILDHOOD CANCER
Gold
COL
D
LEUKEMIA
Orange
LIVER CANCER
Emerald
LUNG CANCER
White
LYMPHOMA
Lime
MELANOMA
Black
MULTIP
B
STOMACH CANCER
Periwinkle
TESTICULAR CANCER
Orchid
THYROID CANCER
Teal/Pink/Blue
UTERINE CANCER
Peach
HONORS CAREGIVERS
Plum
1080154072

CHAPTER 1

Introduction

Felix had been battling cancer for over a year now. He had gone through chemotherapy, radiation, and surgeries, but his body was still weak and constantly fatigued. His doctor had suggested incorporating a healthier diet and juicing into his treatment plan, but Felix had no idea where to start.

One day, as he was scrolling through his social media feed, a sponsored post caught his eye. It was for a book called "Juicing for Cancer Recipes." Intrigued, Felix clicked on the link and read through the reviews.

They were all positive, with many cancer patients raving about the benefits they had experienced from following the recipes in the book.

Without hesitation, Felix ordered the book and eagerly waited for it to arrive.

When it finally arrived in the mail, he tore open the package and dove straight into reading it. The book was beautifully illustrated with colorful pictures of different fruits and vegetables, and it provided a comprehensive guide to juicing for cancer patients. Felix learned about the important nutrients and vitamins found in various fruits and vegetables that could boost his immune system and promote healing in his body. He also discovered specific juice recipes that targeted different symptoms and side effects of cancer treatment, such as nausea, inflammation, and fatigue.

Excited, Felix headed to the grocery store to pick up the ingredients for his first juice recipe, the "Immunity Booster." He followed the instructions in the book and juiced a combination of carrots, apples, ginger, and turmeric. As he took his first sip, he could feel the freshness and nutrients nourishing his body.

Over the next few weeks, Felix tried different juice recipes from the book and noticed a significant improvement in his overall health. His energy levels increased, and he didn't feel as nauseous or fatigued as before. He even shared some of his favorite recipes with his oncologist, who was impressed with the positive changes in Felix's health.

Thanks to "Juicing for Cancer Recipes," Felix was able to incorporate a healthier and more nutritious diet into his cancer treatment plan.

It provided him with a solution to his struggles with maintaining a healthy diet during this challenging time, and he was grateful for the book that had helped him on his journey to recovery.

– Purpose of Juicing for Cancer Recipes Book

The purpose of "Juicing for Cancer Recipes" is to provide cancer patients with a comprehensive guide to incorporating juicing into their treatment plan.

The book offers a variety of nutrient-rich recipes specifically designed for cancer patients, targeting common symptoms and side effects of treatment. Its purpose is to help cancer patients improve their overall health, boost their immune system, and promote healing in their bodies through the power of juicing.

Additionally, the book aims to provide a solution for cancer patients struggling to maintain a healthy diet during their treatment, offering them a convenient and effective way to consume essential vitamins and nutrients.

Ultimately, the purpose of the book is to support and aid in the fight against cancer, providing valuable tools and resources for the journey towards recovery.

– Importance of Nutrition for Cancer Patients

Proper nutrition is crucial for cancer patients as it helps to support their body's ability to fight the disease and manage treatment side effects. Cancer and its treatments can often weaken a person's immune system, making them more susceptible to illnesses and infections.

Therefore, proper nutrition is essential to boost immunity and prevent further health complications. Additionally, a well-balanced and nutritious diet can help patients maintain a healthy weight, which is vital for their recovery and overall health.

Furthermore, certain nutrients found in food can aid in managing treatment side effects such as nausea, fatigue, and inflammation.

For example, ginger and turmeric have anti-inflammatory properties that can help reduce inflammation and pain caused by cancer treatments.

Oranges and leafy greens are rich in vitamin C, which can help reduce nausea and boost the immune system.

Proper nutrition also plays a significant role in supporting the body's recovery process. Cancer treatments can often cause fatigue and weaken the body, making it crucial to consume nutrient-dense foods to aid in the healing process.

Essential vitamins and minerals found in fruits, vegetables, and other whole foods help repair damaged cells and promote cell growth.

In summary, the importance of nutrition for cancer patients cannot be overstated. It is a crucial aspect of their treatment plan, aiding in boosting immunity, managing side effects, and promoting healing. Proper nutrition can significantly impact a person's overall health and well-being during and after their cancer journey.

– Benefits of Juicing for Cancer Patients

Juicing offers numerous benefits for cancer patients, making it a valuable tool to incorporate into their treatment plan.

Firstly, juicing allows patients to easily consume essential vitamins, minerals, and nutrients found in fruits and vegetables. This can be especially beneficial for patients experiencing loss of appetite or difficulty consuming solid foods due to treatment side effects.

Secondly, juicing provides a convenient and efficient way to consume a wide variety of fruits and vegetables. By blending different ingredients together, patients can receive a diverse range of nutrients that may be difficult to obtain through traditional meals.

This is particularly important for cancer patients as they require a well-balanced diet to support their recovery and fight the disease.

Moreover, the high concentration of nutrients in juices can help boost the immune system and aid in the body's healing process. Many fruits and vegetables contain antioxidants and anti-inflammatory properties that can help reduce inflammation and support the body's natural defenses.

Additionally, juicing is a great way to manage common treatment side effects such as nausea and fatigue. By targeting specific symptoms, juicing recipes can provide relief and help patients feel more energized and comfortable.

Lastly, juicing can also serve as a source of hydration for cancer patients. Staying hydrated is crucial for patients undergoing treatment as it helps flush out toxins and keep the body functioning properly.

In conclusion, the benefits of juicing for cancer patients are numerous, making it an excellent addition to their treatment plan. From boosting immunity to managing side effects, juicing can play a significant role in supporting patients' overall health and well-being during their journey to recovery.

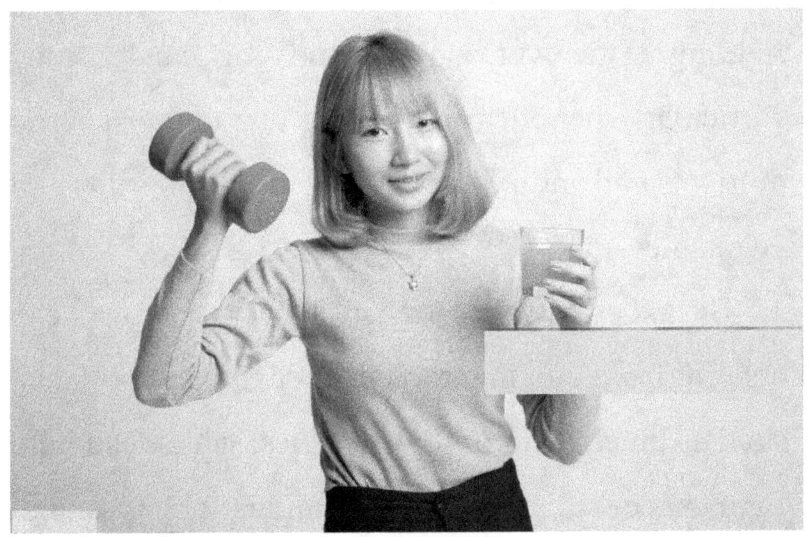

CHAPTER II. UNDERSTANDING CANCER AND ITS TREATMENT

– Different Types of Cancer

Juicing can benefit cancer patients of all types, regardless of the specific type of cancer they are fighting. However, some types of cancer may particularly benefit from juicing due to the specific nutrients and antioxidants found in certain fruits and vegetables.

1. Breast Cancer: Breast cancer patients can benefit from juicing recipes rich in antioxidants, such as blueberries and raspberries, which can help fight cancer cells. Additionally, juicing recipes high in vitamin C, like citrus fruits, can help improve the effectiveness of chemotherapy.

2. Prostate Cancer: Cruciferous vegetables like broccoli, cauliflower, and kale have been shown to have anti-cancer properties that may be beneficial for prostate cancer patients. These vegetables are often used in juicing recipes and can help reduce inflammation and promote healing.

3. Lung Cancer: Many juicing recipes contain ginger, which has anti-inflammatory properties that can help manage lung cancer symptoms such as coughing and difficulty breathing. Juicing recipes high in vitamin C, like oranges and red peppers, may also aid in reducing lung cancer risk.

4. Colon Cancer: Colon cancer patients can benefit from consuming juicing recipes rich in fiber, like apples, beets, and leafy greens. Fiber can help keep the digestive system healthy and alleviate constipation, a common side effect of colon cancer treatments.

5. Blood Cancer: Blood cancers, such as leukemia and lymphoma, can benefit from juicing recipes high in iron, folate, and B vitamins, like spinach and beets. These nutrients can help support the production of healthy blood cells and improve overall energy levels.

In summary, juicing can benefit cancer patients of all types, but specific types of cancer may benefit from ingredients and nutrients found in certain fruits and vegetables.

It is essential for patients to consult with their doctor and tailor juicing recipes to their specific needs and treatment plan.

- Common Cancer Treatment Methods

There are several common treatment methods for cancer, including chemotherapy, radiation, and surgery. Each of these treatments can have various side effects, such as nausea, fatigue, and inflammation.

Juicing can be a helpful addition to a cancer patient's treatment plan, as it provides essential vitamins and nutrients to support the body's healing process and alleviate treatment side effects.

Chemotherapy: Chemotherapy works by killing rapidly dividing cancer cells, but it can also damage healthy cells, leading to side effects such as nausea, loss of appetite, and fatigue. Juicing can help cancer patients stay hydrated and provide nutrients to support their body's recovery. Ginger, peppermint, and apple juice are commonly recommended for nausea relief.

Radiation: Radiation therapy targets and kills cancer cells in a specific area, but it can also damage healthy cells and cause various side effects, including inflammation and skin irritation. Juicing recipes high in antioxidants, such as blueberries and cherries, can help reduce inflammation and promote healing.

Surgery: Surgery involves removing cancerous tumors and tissues from the body, which can be physically and emotionally taxing for patients.

Proper nutrition is crucial to support the body's recovery and healing post-surgery.

Juicing recipes high in protein, such as almond milk and Greek yogurt, can help with the recovery process.

In conclusion, juicing can be beneficial for cancer patients undergoing different treatment methods. It can help manage treatment side effects, provide essential nutrients for the body's healing process, and aid in recovery post-surgery.

It is important for patients to consult with their doctors and tailor juicing recipes to their specific needs and treatment plan.

- Nutritional Challenges During Cancer Treatment

Cancer treatment can be physically and emotionally taxing, and patients often face nutritional challenges that can further affect their health. Some common nutritional challenges during cancer treatment include loss of appetite, difficulty eating solid foods, and weight loss.

Juicing can help overcome these challenges by providing patients with easily digestible nutrients and promoting a diverse, nutrient-rich diet.

Loss of Appetite: Many cancer patients experience a loss of appetite due to their illness or treatment. Consuming large quantities of whole foods may be challenging, but juicing offers a solution by providing a concentrated dose of essential vitamins and minerals in a less intimidating form.

Difficulty Eating Solid Foods: Some cancer treatments can cause difficulty eating solid foods due to mouth pain, sore throat, or difficulty swallowing. Juicing allows patients to receive the necessary nutrients without causing additional pain or discomfort.

Weight Loss: Some cancer treatments can cause patients to lose weight as a side effect. Juicing provides a convenient and efficient way to consume nutrient-dense foods and helps patients maintain healthy weight levels.

In conclusion, juicing can be a valuable tool for cancer patients facing nutritional challenges during treatment.

It provides a solution for patients experiencing loss of appetite or difficulty consuming solid foods while also promoting a balanced and diverse diet. Juicing can help support overall health and well-being during the cancer journey.

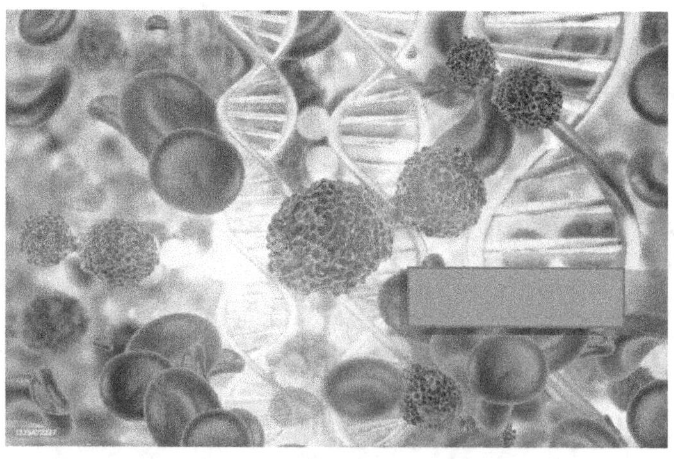

CHAPTER III. JUICING BASICS

- Importance of Fresh Fruits and Vegetables

The importance of using fresh fruits and vegetables in juicing for cancer patients cannot be emphasized enough. Fresh produce is bursting with essential vitamins, minerals, and antioxidants that are vital for the body's healing and recovery process.

When fruits and vegetables are juiced, their nutrients are in a concentrated form and are easily absorbed by the body, making fresh produce a crucial element in juicing for cancer patients.

Furthermore, fresh fruits and vegetables are free of preservatives, additives, and chemicals, making them a healthier option for cancer patients who need to consume nutrient-dense, natural foods. Consuming too many processed foods can weaken the body's immune system, making it harder for patients to fight the disease.

Moreover, fresh fruits and vegetables offer a diverse range of nutrients that are necessary for a well-balanced diet.

Juicing with a variety of produce can provide patients with a wide range of vitamins and minerals that may be difficult to obtain through regular meals.

Fresh fruits and vegetables also help keep the body hydrated, which is crucial for cancer patients undergoing treatment. Proper hydration can help flush out toxins and support the body's natural defenses, aiding in the healing process.

In conclusion, fresh fruits and vegetables are essential for juicing for cancer patients as they provide necessary nutrients, are free from harmful additives, and aid in hydration.

It is important for patients to incorporate a variety of fresh produce into their juicing recipes for optimal health benefits.

– Choosing the Right Juicer

Choosing the right juicer is an essential factor to consider when juicing for cancer patients. There are a variety of juicers on the market, each with different features and capabilities.

When selecting a juicer for a cancer patient, it is crucial to consider their individual needs and treatment plan.

For patients with weakened immune systems, a juicer with easy-clean features may be beneficial as it can prevent the growth of harmful bacteria on the juicer's components.

Similarly, juicers that have a pulp-ejecting feature may be more convenient for patients experiencing fatigue as it eliminates the need to empty the pulp collector repeatedly.

Patients undergoing chemotherapy may benefit from using a juicer with slow-press technology, as it minimizes heat production and oxidation, preserving the nutrients in the juice. This is especially important for cancer patients as they require a higher concentration of nutrients to support their body's healing and recovery.

Additionally, cancer patients with mouth or throat pain may find it helpful to choose a juicer with an additional strainer, resulting in a smoother juice with less pulp.

In conclusion, choosing the right juicer is crucial for cancer patients as it can affect the quality and nutrient content of their juice.

With proper research and consideration of individual needs, the right juicer can significantly enhance the benefits of juicing for cancer patients.

– Preparation and Storage of Produce

Preparation and storage of produce is a crucial step in juicing for cancer patients to ensure the safety and quality of the juice. Proper cleaning and handling of fruits and vegetables can prevent the growth of harmful bacteria, which can be dangerous for patients with weakened immune systems.

Before juicing, it is important to thoroughly wash all produce, even if it has been pre-washed. This removes any potential dirt, bacteria, or pesticides that may be on the surface.

Scrubbing with a vegetable brush under running water is recommended for leafy greens and firm fruits and vegetables.

Proper storage of produce is also essential to maintain its freshness and nutritional value. Fruits and vegetables should be stored in the refrigerator, preferably in a crisper drawer, to keep them cool and crisp until juicing.

Produce should also be stored separately, as certain fruits, such as apples, bananas, and avocado, emit ethylene gas that can cause other fruits and vegetables to ripen and spoil faster.

It is also important to monitor produce for any signs of spoilage before juicing.

In conclusion, proper preparation and storage of produce is vital in juicing for cancer patients to maintain the safety and quality of juice.

By following these guidelines, cancer patients can safely and confidently consume nutrient-rich juices as part of their treatment plan.

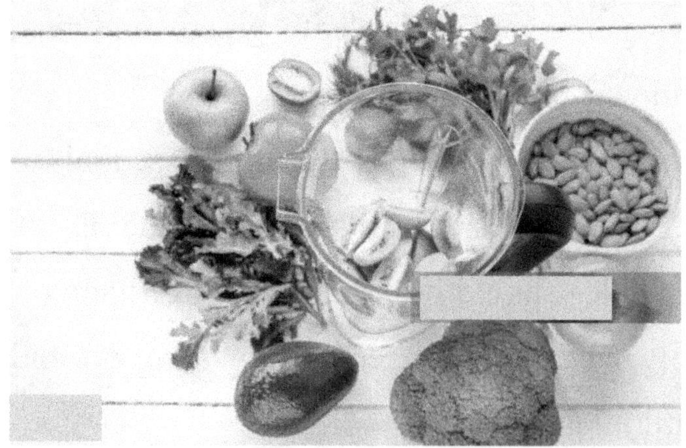

CHAPTER IV. ANTI-CANCER INGREDIENTS

– Fruits and Vegetables with Anti-Cancer Properties

There are many fruits and vegetables with anti-cancer properties that can be beneficial for cancer patients when juiced. Incorporating these ingredients into juicing recipes can provide patients with a concentrated dose of essential vitamins, minerals, and antioxidants, which are crucial for supporting the body's healing and recovery process.

1. Berry fruits: Berries, such as blueberries, raspberries, and strawberries, are rich in polyphenols, which have been shown to have anti-cancer properties. These fruits are also high in antioxidants, making them a beneficial addition to juicing recipes for cancer patients.

2. Cruciferous vegetables: Vegetables like broccoli, cauliflower, and kale contain compounds that have been linked to a lower risk of cancer. They are also high in fiber, which can aid in digestion and help maintain a healthy colon.

3. Citrus fruits: Citrus fruits like oranges, lemons, and grapefruits are high in vitamin C, which has been shown to help boost the immune system and improve the effectiveness of chemotherapy.

These fruits also contain antioxidants and anti-inflammatory properties.

4. Leafy greens: Leafy greens, such as spinach, kale, and collard greens, are packed with beneficial nutrients such as vitamin C, fiber, and folate. They have also been linked to a lower risk of certain types of cancer.

5. Turmeric: Turmeric has anti-inflammatory properties and is commonly used in juicing recipes for cancer patients to aid in reducing inflammation and promoting healing.

In conclusion, incorporating these fruits and vegetables with anti-cancer properties into juicing recipes can provide cancer patients with a concentrated dose of essential nutrients and antioxidants to support their body's healing and recovery.

It is essential to consult with a healthcare professional before making any significant changes to a patient's diet or juicing routine.

– How to Incorporate Juicing into a Cancer Treatment Plan

Incorporating juicing into a cancer treatment plan can provide numerous benefits for patients, including boosting immunity, managing treatment side effects, and promoting healing. However, it is crucial to consult with a healthcare professional before making any significant changes to a treatment plan.

Here are some tips on how to safely and effectively incorporate juicing into a cancer treatment plan.

1. Talk to the doctor: Before starting any juicing regimen, it is important to speak with the doctor to ensure it is safe and suitable for an individual's specific treatment plan. Some treatment methods and medications may interact with certain fruits and vegetables, so it is crucial to get professional advice.

2. Use fresh produce: When juicing for cancer patients, it is important to use fresh and clean produce. This ensures the safety of the juice and provides maximum nutritional value.

3. Choose appropriate ingredients: Certain fruits and vegetables may be more beneficial for specific types of cancer or treatment side effects. For example, ginger is known to alleviate nausea, while leafy greens aid in digestion.

Consult with a healthcare professional or do research to choose ingredients that cater to an individual's needs.

4. Slowly incorporate into the diet: Patients should slowly incorporate juicing into their diet to prevent any adverse reactions. Gradually increasing the frequency and portion sizes of juices can also help the body adjust to the change.

5. Monitor for any negative reactions: After incorporating juicing into a treatment plan, it is important to monitor for any negative reactions or interactions. If any symptoms arise, consult with a healthcare professional immediately.

In conclusion, incorporating juicing into a cancer treatment plan requires proper preparation, monitoring, and consultation with a healthcare professional.

By taking these precautions, patients can safely and effectively reap the benefits of juicing as part of their journey towards recovery.

- Superfoods for Cancer Patients

Including superfoods in juicing recipes can provide cancer patients with a concentrated dose of essential nutrients, antioxidants, and anti-inflammatory compounds. These powerful ingredients can help support the body's healing and recovery process. Here are some superfoods that can be incorporated into juicing recipes for cancer patients.

1. Turmeric: This bright yellow spice has anti-inflammatory and antioxidant properties, and is commonly used in juicing to help reduce inflammation and promote healing.

2. Cruciferous vegetables: These include vegetables like broccoli, cauliflower, and Brussels sprouts, which contain compounds linked to a lower risk of cancer. They are also high in fiber, which can aid in digestion and help maintain a healthy colon.

3. Berries: Berries such as blueberries, strawberries, and raspberries are packed with antioxidants and polyphenols, which have been shown to have anti-cancer properties.

4. Leafy greens: Leafy greens, including spinach, kale, and collard greens, are rich in beneficial nutrients such as fiber, vitamin C, and folate, and have been linked to a lower risk of certain types of cancer.

5. Ginger: Ginger has anti-inflammatory properties and is commonly used in juicing to help alleviate nausea, which is a common side effect of cancer treatment.

6. Citrus fruits: Citrus fruits like lemons, oranges, and grapefruits are high in vitamin C and antioxidants, and can help boost the immune system and improve the effectiveness of chemotherapy.

7. Avocado: Avocados are a good source of healthy fats and are rich in antioxidants and anti-inflammatory compounds.

They can also help improve nutrient absorption and promote healing.

In conclusion, incorporating these superfoods into juicing recipes can provide cancer patients with a variety of beneficial nutrients that can support their healing and recovery.

It is important to consult with a healthcare professional before making any significant changes to an individual's diet or juicing routine.

- Herbs and Spices for Boosting Immunity

Incorporating herbs and spices into juicing recipes can provide cancer patients with a powerful boost of nutrients and immune-boosting properties. These ingredients can help support the body's natural defenses and aid in the healing and recovery process.

Here are some herbs and spices to consider including in juicing recipes for cancer patients.

1. Ginger: Ginger has anti-inflammatory and antioxidant properties, making it a popular ingredient in juicing to help reduce inflammation and promote healing. It is also commonly used to alleviate nausea, a common side effect of cancer treatment.

2. Turmeric: This golden spice has potent anti-inflammatory and antioxidant properties, making it a powerful ally for cancer patients. Incorporating it into juicing can help reduce inflammation and support the body's healing process.

3. Garlic: Garlic has antibacterial, anti-inflammatory, and immune-boosting properties, making it a valuable addition to juicing recipes for cancer patients. Its sulfur-containing compounds may also play a role in cancer prevention.

4. Basil: This flavorful herb is packed with immune-boosting vitamins and minerals, including vitamin C, calcium, and magnesium. Additionally, it might be antibacterial and anti-inflammatory.

5. Cinnamon: This warm spice is rich in antioxidants and has been shown to have anti-inflammatory and antimicrobial properties. It can enhance general health and wellbeing and assist the immune system.

6. Oregano: Oregano is a good source of vitamins and minerals, including vitamin K, manganese, and iron. It also contains powerful antioxidants and may have anti-inflammatory and antibacterial properties. In conclusion, incorporating these herbs and spices into juicing recipes can provide cancer patients with a boost of immune-boosting nutrients and compounds.

It is important to consult with a healthcare professional before making any significant changes to a treatment plan or diet.

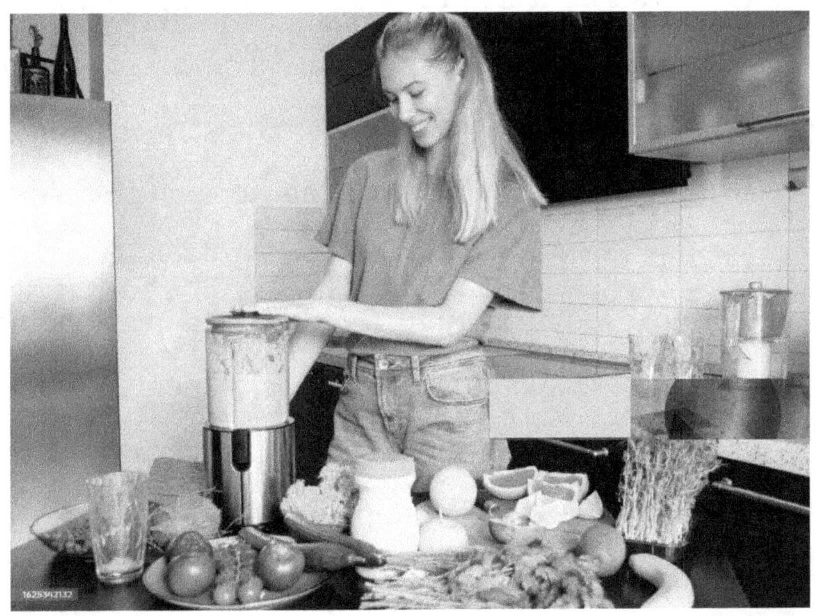

CHAPTER V. JUICING RECIPES FOR COMMON CANCER SYMPTOMS

- Nausea and Vomiting

Juicing can be a helpful way to manage common cancer symptoms such as nausea and vomiting. Certain ingredients can soothe the stomach and provide a concentrated dose of nutrients in an easily digestible form.

Here are some juicing recipes that may help alleviate these symptoms for cancer patients.

1. Ginger and Carrot Juice: Ginger has been shown to have anti-inflammatory and anti-nausea properties, making it a popular ingredient for nausea-relief. Combining it with vitamin-rich carrots can provide a powerful boost of nutrients for cancer patients.

Simply juice 1-2 inches of fresh ginger root with 3-4 medium sized carrots for a soothing and nutritious drink.

2. Green Power Juice: This juice combines leafy greens, cucumber, and lemon to create a refreshing and nutrient-packed drink. The high water content in cucumber can help hydrate and soothe the stomach, while lemon provides a dose of vitamin C to boost the immune system. Juice 1 cup of kale, 1 peeled cucumber, and 1 lemon (peeled).

3. Banana and Blueberry Smoothie: If solid foods are difficult to tolerate, a smoothie may be a better option. This recipe combines anti-inflammatory blueberries with fiber-rich banana for a nutritious and filling drink. Simply blend 1 cup of frozen blueberries with 1 ripe banana and 1 cup of your choice of milk (dairy, almond, soy, etc.).

4. Peppermint Tea Infused Juice: Peppermint has been used for centuries for its calming and digestion-promoting properties. You can infuse these benefits into a juice by steeping a peppermint tea bag in a cup of hot water for 3-5 minutes. Let the tea cool, then use it as a base for your favorite juice recipe, like a green juice or carrot juice.

Always consult with a healthcare professional before incorporating juicing into a cancer treatment plan. These recipes are meant to provide guidance and inspiration, but individual needs and sensitivities may vary.

- Loss of Appetite

Loss of appetite is a common symptom among cancer patients, and it can be challenging to maintain a well-balanced diet. Juicing can provide a convenient and nutritious way to still consume essential nutrients and promote healing. Here are some juicing recipes that may help boost appetite and provide vital nutrients for cancer patients.

1. Avocado Smoothie: Avocado is a great source of healthy fats and essential nutrients, making it a nourishing addition to a juice or smoothie. This recipe blends ½ an avocado with 1 cup of your choice of milk (dairy, almond, soy, etc.) and a handful of spinach. It can be sweetened with honey or maple syrup if desired.

2. Creamy Berry Juice: Berries are full of antioxidants and essential nutrients, making them a great ingredient for a nutritious juice. This recipe combines 1 cup of your choice of frozen berries with 1 cup of Greek yogurt and ½ a cup of milk. It can be sweetened with honey if desired.

3. Sweet Potato Juice: Sweet potatoes are high in nutrients and have a naturally sweet flavor, making them a great choice for a juice. Juice 1 medium-sized sweet potato to create a rich and nutritious drink.

4. Beet and Apple Juice: Beets are packed with essential vitamins and minerals, and their natural sweetness can help make this juice more palatable for cancer patients with a loss of appetite. Juice 1 small beet with 1-2 apples for a refreshing and nutrient-dense drink.

Always consult with a healthcare professional before incorporating juicing into a cancer treatment plan. These recipes are meant to provide guidance and inspiration, but individual needs and sensitivities may vary.

- Digestive Issues

Digestive issues are a common side effect of cancer treatment, and juicing can be a helpful way to support and soothe the digestive system. Certain ingredients can provide a boost of nutrients and compounds to promote healing and alleviate discomfort. Here are some juicing recipes that may help manage digestive issues for cancer patients.

1. Pineapple Spinach Juice: Pineapple contains an enzyme called bromelain, which has been shown to aid in digestion and reduce inflammation. Combining it with nutrient-rich spinach makes for a powerful drink for supporting digestive health. Juice 1 cup of fresh or frozen pineapple with 1 cup of spinach for a refreshing and nutritious drink.

2. Cucumber, Ginger, and Lemon Juice: Cucumber has a high water content and can help soothe the stomach, while ginger and lemon have anti-inflammatory properties. Combine these ingredients for a powerful digestive aid. Juice 1 peeled cucumber, 2 inches of fresh ginger root, and 1 lemon (peeled).

3. Papaya and Banana Smoothie: Papaya contains a digestive enzyme called papain, which can help break down protein and aid in digestion. Combine this with potassium-rich banana in a smoothie for a nutritious and easy-to-digest drink. Blend 1 cup of fresh or frozen papaya with 1 ripe banana and 1 cup of your choice of milk (dairy, almond, soy, etc.).

4. Carrot and Celery Juice: Carrots are rich in essential nutrients that can support digestive health, while celery has anti-inflammatory properties. Juice 3-4 medium-sized carrots with 2-3 celery stalks for a nutrient-dense drink.

Always consult with a healthcare professional before incorporating juicing into a cancer treatment plan.

These recipes are meant to provide guidance and inspiration, but individual needs and sensitivities may vary.

- Fatigue

Fatigue is a common symptom for cancer patients, and it can be challenging to find the energy to consume nutritious meals. Juicing can provide a convenient way to consume essential vitamins and minerals that can help support energy levels and promote healing. Here are some juicing recipes that may provide a boost of energy for cancer patients dealing with fatigue.

1. Green Power Juice: This juice combines nutrient-dense leafy greens and hydrating cucumber to create a refreshing and energizing drink. Juice 1 cup of kale, 1 peeled cucumber, and 1 lemon (peeled) for a nutrient-packed and hydrating drink.

2. Carrot and Beet Juice: Carrots and beets are both rich in essential vitamins and minerals, making them a great energy-boosting combination. Juice 3-4 medium-sized carrots with 1 small beet for a sweet and nutritious drink.

3. Energizing Berry Smoothie: Berries are a great source of antioxidants and can provide a powerful boost of energy for cancer patients. Blend 1 cup of your choice of frozen berries with 1 banana and 1 cup of your choice of milk (dairy, almond, soy, etc.) for a refreshing and energizing smoothie.

4. Orange and Ginger Juice: Oranges are high in vitamin C and have energizing properties, while ginger provides anti-inflammatory benefits. Juice 2-3 oranges with 1-2 inches of fresh ginger root for a zesty and nutrient-rich drink.

Always consult with a healthcare professional before incorporating juicing into a cancer treatment plan.

These recipes are meant to provide guidance and inspiration, but individual needs and sensitivities may vary.

– Insomnia

Insomnia can be a challenging symptom for cancer patients, and it can greatly impact overall well-being and recovery. Certain juicing recipes can help promote sleep and relaxation, providing a natural way to combat insomnia.

Here are some juicing recipes to consider for cancer patients struggling with insomnia.

1. **Golden Milk Juice:** This juice combines soothing and sleep-promoting ingredients like

turmeric, ginger, and milk. Juice 1-2 inches of fresh ginger root with ½-1 teaspoon of turmeric powder and 1 cup of your choice of milk (dairy, almond, soy, etc.).

2. Chamomile and Berry Smoothie: Chamomile tea is known for its sleep-promoting properties, and it can be infused into a smoothie for a nutritious and calming drink. Infuse a chamomile tea bag in a cup of hot water for 3-5 minutes, then let it cool. Blend the tea with 1 cup of your choice of frozen berries and 1 banana for a delicious and soothing drink.

3. Banana and Honey Juice: Bananas contain high levels of the amino acid tryptophan, which can promote relaxation and sleep. Combined with honey, which has been shown to improve sleep quality, this juice may help combat insomnia. Juice 1-2 ripe bananas with a teaspoon of honey for a sweet and sleep-promoting drink.

4. Lavender and Lemon Juice: Lavender has been used for centuries for its calming and sleep-promoting properties, making it a valuable ingredient for a juice. Steep a lavender tea bag in a cup of hot water for 3-5 minutes, then let it cool. Juice 1 lemon and combine it with the tea for a refreshing and sleep-promoting drink.

Always consult with a healthcare professional before incorporating juicing into a cancer treatment plan. These recipes are meant to provide guidance and inspiration, but individual needs and sensitivities may vary.

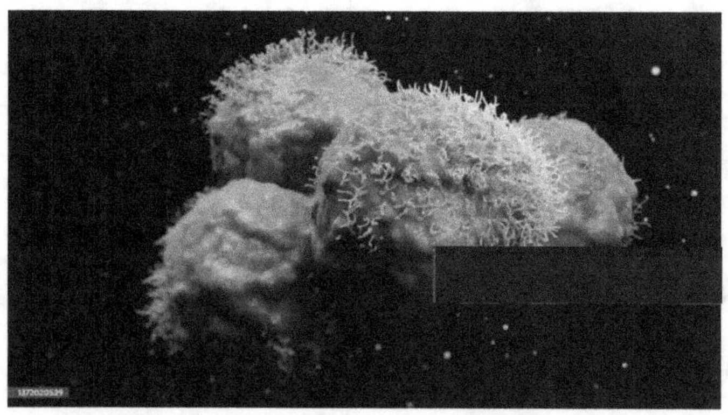

CHAPTER VI. JUICING RECIPES FOR SPECIFIC TYPES OF CANCER

- Breast Cancer

Breast cancer is a complex disease, and a nutritious diet can play a crucial role in supporting treatment and recovery. Certain juicing recipes may provide essential nutrients and antioxidants that can help fight cancer cells and promote overall health. Here are some juicing recipes to consider for breast cancer patients.

1. Broccoli and Orange Juice: Broccoli is a cruciferous vegetable that contains beneficial compounds that may help lower the risk of breast cancer. Combined with high levels of vitamin C in oranges, this juice can provide a powerful dose of cancer-fighting nutrients. Juice 1 cup of broccoli with 2-3 oranges for a nutritious and anti-cancer drink.

2. Pomegranate and Beet Juice: Pomegranates are rich in antioxidants and have been shown to have anti-cancer properties. Combined with the high levels of folate in beets, this juice may help protect against breast cancer. Juice 1 pomegranate with 1 small beet for a sweet and potentially cancer-fighting drink.

3. Kale and Berry Smoothie: Kale is a nutrient-dense leafy green that contains compounds that may help protect against breast cancer. Combined with antioxidant-rich berries, this smoothie can provide a powerful dose of cancer-fighting nutrients. Blend 1 cup of kale with 1 cup of your choice of frozen berries and 1 banana for a delicious and nutritious drink.

4. Turmeric and Ginger Shot: Turmeric and ginger both contain anti-inflammatory and antioxidant properties that may help prevent breast cancer. Combined in a potent shot, they can provide a powerful dose of cancer-fighting nutrients. Juice 1-2 inches of fresh ginger root with ½-1 teaspoon of turmeric powder for a zesty and anti-cancer shot.

Always consult with a healthcare professional before incorporating juicing into a breast cancer treatment plan. These recipes are meant to provide guidance and inspiration, but individual needs and sensitivities may vary.

- Lung Cancer

Lung cancer can be a challenging disease to manage, and a nutritious diet can play a significant role in supporting treatment and recovery. Certain juicing recipes may provide essential nutrients and antioxidants that can help fight cancer cells and promote lung health. Here are some juicing recipes to consider for lung cancer patients.

1. Carrot and Ginger Juice: Carrots and ginger are both high in antioxidants and anti-inflammatory compounds that can help protect against lung cancer. Juice 3-4 medium-sized carrots with 1-2 inches of fresh ginger root for a refreshing and potentially cancer-fighting drink.

2. Blueberry and Spinach Smoothie: Blueberries are packed with antioxidants and have been shown to have anti-cancer properties. Combined with nutrient-dense spinach, this smoothie can provide a potent dose of cancer-fighting nutrients. Blend 1 cup of blueberries with a handful of spinach and 1 cup of your choice of milk (dairy, almond, soy, etc.) for a delicious and potentially lung-protective drink.

3. Garlic and Lemon Shot: Garlic contains compounds that have been shown to have anti-cancer properties, and lemon is high in vitamin C and may help protect against lung cancer. Combined in a potent shot, these ingredients can provide a powerful dose of cancer-fighting nutrients. Juice 1-2 cloves of garlic with 1 lemon for a potent and potentially lung-protective shot.

4. Grapefruit and Beet Juice: Grapefruit is high in antioxidants and has been shown to have anti-cancer properties. Combined with the high levels of folate in beets, this juice may help protect against lung cancer. Juice 1 grapefruit with 1 small beet for a tangy and potentially cancer-fighting drink.

Always consult with a healthcare professional before incorporating juicing into a lung cancer treatment plan. These recipes are meant to provide guidance and inspiration, but individual needs and sensitivities may vary.

- Prostate Cancer

Prostate cancer is a significant health concern for men, and a nutritious diet can play a crucial role in supporting treatment and recovery. Certain juicing recipes may provide essential nutrients and antioxidants that can help fight cancer cells and promote prostate health. Here are some juicing recipes to consider for prostate cancer patients.

1. Tomato and Celery Juice: Tomatoes are high in lycopene, a compound with powerful anti-cancer properties, and celery contains anti-inflammatory compounds that may help protect against prostate cancer. Juice 1-2 large tomatoes with 2-3 stalks of celery for a tangy and potentially cancer-fighting drink.

2. Green Tea and Mango Smoothie: Green tea is packed with antioxidants and has been shown to have anti-cancer properties. Combined with the anti-inflammatory and antioxidant benefits of mangoes, this smoothie can provide a potent dose of cancer-fighting nutrients. Brew 1 cup of green tea and let it cool.

Blend the tea with 1 cup of frozen mango and 1 banana for a refreshing and potentially prostate-protective drink.

3. Watermelon and Mint Juice: Watermelon is high in lycopene and has been associated with a lower risk of prostate cancer. Combined with the calming and anti-inflammatory benefits of mint, this juice may help protect against prostate cancer. Juice 1-2 cups of watermelon with a handful of mint leaves for a refreshing and potentially cancer-fighting drink.

4. Pineapple and Ginger Shot: Pineapple contains bromelain, an enzyme known for its anti-inflammatory properties, and ginger has been shown to have anti-cancer effects. Combined in a potent shot, these ingredients can provide a powerful dose of cancer-fighting nutrients. Juice 1 cup of pineapple with 1-2 inches of fresh ginger root for a potent and potentially prostate-protective shot. Always consult with a healthcare professional before incorporating juicing into a prostate cancer treatment plan. These recipes are meant to provide guidance and inspiration, but individual needs and sensitivities may vary.

Colon cancer can be a challenging disease to manage, and a nutritious diet can play a significant role in supporting treatment and recovery. Certain juicing recipes may provide essential nutrients and antioxidants that can help fight cancer cells and promote colon health. Here are some juicing recipes to consider for colon cancer patients.

1. Spinach and Kiwi Juice: Spinach is a nutrient-dense leafy green that contains compounds that may help protect against colon cancer. Combined with the high levels of vitamin C in kiwis, this juice can provide a powerful dose of cancer-fighting nutrients.

Juice a handful of spinach with 2-3 ripe kiwis for a refreshing and potentially cancer-fighting drink.

2. Blackberry and Mint Smoothie: Blackberries are high in antioxidants and have been shown to have anti-cancer properties. Combined with the calming and anti-inflammatory benefits of mint, this smoothie can provide a potent dose of cancer-fighting nutrients.

Blend 1 cup of blackberries with a handful of mint leaves and 1 cup of your choice of milk (dairy, almond, soy, etc.) for a delicious and potentially colon-protective drink.

3. Beet and Carrot Juice: Beets are high in folate and contain compounds that may help lower the risk of colon cancer. Combined with the anti-inflammatory and antioxidant benefits of carrots, this juice can provide a powerful defense against colon cancer.

Juice 1 small beet with 3-4 medium-sized carrots for a sweet and potentially cancer-fighting drink.

4. Turmeric and Lemon Shot: Turmeric contains curcumin, a compound with potent anti-cancer properties, and lemon is high in vitamin C and may help protect against colon cancer. Combined in a potent shot, these ingredients can provide a powerful dose of cancer-fighting nutrients.

Juice 1-2 inches of fresh turmeric root with 1 lemon for a zesty and potentially colon-protective shot.

Always consult with a healthcare professional before incorporating juicing into a colon cancer treatment plan. These recipes are meant to provide guidance and inspiration, but individual needs and sensitivities may vary.

- Leukemia

Leukemia is a complex and challenging disease, and a nutritious diet can play a crucial role in supporting treatment and recovery.

Certain juicing recipes may provide essential nutrients and antioxidants that can help fight cancer cells and promote overall health. Here are some juicing recipes to consider for leukemia patients.

1. Kale and Pineapple Juice: Kale is a nutrient-dense leafy green that contains compounds that may help protect against leukemia. Combined with the high levels of vitamin C and bromelain in pineapples, this juice can provide a powerful dose of cancer-fighting nutrients. Juice 1 cup of kale with 1 cup of pineapple for a refreshing and potentially cancer-fighting drink.

2. Blueberry and Ginger Smoothie: Blueberries are packed with antioxidants and have been shown to have anti-cancer properties. Combined with the anti-inflammatory and immune-boosting benefits of ginger, this smoothie can provide a potent dose of cancer-fighting nutrients.

Blend 1 cup of blueberries with 1-2 inches of fresh ginger root and 1 cup of your choice of milk (dairy, almond, soy, etc.) for a delicious and potentially leukemia-fighting drink.

3. Turmeric and Carrot Juice: Turmeric contains curcumin, a compound with potent anti-cancer properties, and carrots contain beneficial nutrients and antioxidants. Combined in a juice, these ingredients can provide a powerful defense against leukemia.

Juice 1-2 inches of fresh turmeric root with 3-4 medium-sized carrots for a nutrient-dense and potentially cancer-fighting drink.

4. Orange and Mango Shot: Oranges are high in antioxidants and have been shown to have anti-cancer effects, while mangoes are rich in beneficial nutrients and enzymes. Combined in a potent shot, these ingredients can provide a powerful dose of cancer-fighting nutrients.

Juice 1 orange with 1 cup of ripe mango for a potent and potentially leukemia-fighting shot.

Always consult with a healthcare professional before incorporating juicing into a leukemia treatment plan. These recipes are meant to provide guidance and inspiration, but individual needs and sensitivities may vary.

CHAPTER VII. JUICING FOR CANCER PREVENTION

– Lifestyle and Dietary Factors for Prevention

Cancer is a complex disease, and while there is no single factor that can prevent it, certain lifestyle and dietary habits may help reduce the risk. Here are some key lifestyle and dietary factors to consider for cancer prevention:

1. Maintain a healthy weight: Being overweight or obese can increase the risk of various types of cancer. By maintaining a healthy weight and body mass index (BMI), you may lower your risk of developing cancer.

2. Limit alcohol consumption: Excessive alcohol consumption has been linked to an increased risk of various types of cancer, including breast, liver, and colorectal cancer. Limiting your alcohol intake or avoiding it altogether can help reduce the risk.

3. Quit smoking: Tobacco use is one of the leading causes of cancer, and quitting smoking is one of the most effective ways to prevent it. It might also lessen the chance of a cancer relapse.

4. Consume a diet rich in fruits and vegetables: A diet high in fruits and vegetables provides essential vitamins, minerals, and antioxidants that may help protect against cancer. Aim for a variety of colors and types of produce to ensure a well-rounded intake of nutrients.

5. Limit processed and red meat consumption: Eating too much processed or red meat has been linked to an increased risk of colorectal cancer.

Aim to limit your intake and incorporate more plant-based proteins in your diet.

6. Exercise regularly: Regular physical activity can help maintain a healthy weight and may decrease the risk of certain types of cancer. Aim for at least 30 minutes of moderate activity, such as walking or jogging, each day.

7. Limit exposure to harmful substances: Exposure to certain chemicals and substances, such as asbestos and UV rays, can increase the risk of cancer. Take protective measures and limit your exposure to these harmful substances.

In addition to these lifestyle and dietary factors, following a regular healthcare routine and undergoing recommended screenings can also play a crucial role in preventing cancer.

Never forget to seek the counsel and recommendations of a healthcare professional for individualised advice.

– Juicing Recipes for a Healthy and Balanced Diet

Juicing is a popular way to incorporate more fruits and vegetables into your diet and reap the numerous health benefits they offer. Here are some juicing recipes to help you maintain a healthy and balanced diet:

1. Green Goddess Juice: This juice is packed with greens and other nutritious ingredients, making it an excellent way to start your day. Juice 1 green apple, 1 cup of spinach, 1 cucumber, 1 lemon, and 1-inch piece of ginger for a refreshing and nutrient-dense drink.

2. Sunshine Smoothie: This bright and vibrant smoothie is loaded with Vitamin C and other beneficial nutrients. Blend 1 cup of frozen mango, 1 cup of orange juice, 1 banana, and 1 small carrot for a delicious and nutritious drink.

3. Antioxidant Blast Juice: This juice is packed with antioxidants, which may help protect against various diseases. Juice 1 cup of blueberries, 1 small beet, 1 large carrot, and 1 inch of fresh ginger for a nutritious and potentially disease-fighting drink.

4. Protein-Packed Green Juice: This juice provides a boost of protein, making it an excellent post-workout drink or a satisfying meal replacement.

Juice 1 small green apple, 1 cup of kale, 1/2 avocado, 1/4 cup of protein powder, and 1 cup of almond milk for a filling and nutrient-dense drink.

Remember to incorporate these juices into a well-balanced diet that includes a variety of other whole foods.

Consult with a healthcare professional for personalized recommendations on how to incorporate juicing into your diet for optimal health and wellness.

- Incorporating Juicing into Daily Routine

Juicing can be a beneficial addition to your daily routine, providing a quick and convenient way to consume essential vitamins, minerals, and antioxidants.

Here are some tips on how to incorporate juicing into your daily routine for maximum benefits:

1. Start your day with a juice or smoothie: Starting your day with a nutritious juice or smoothie is a great way to kickstart your metabolism and provide your body with a boost of vitamins and minerals.

2. Use juicing as a snack or meal replacement: Rather than reaching for a sugary or processed snack, opt for a nutrient-dense juice or smoothie as a healthy snack. You can also replace one meal per day with a juice or smoothie, but remember to incorporate other whole foods into your diet as well.

3. Experiment with different ingredients: Don't be afraid to try new and unique combinations of ingredients in your juices and smoothies. This will not only provide a variety of nutrients but also keep your taste buds excited.

4. Pre-prepare ingredients: To save time, pre-prepare your ingredients by washing, cutting, and storing them in the fridge or freezer. This way, you can quickly make a juice or smoothie without the hassle of preparing each ingredient every time.

5. Make it a family affair: Juicing can be a fun family activity. Involve your children or other family members in the juicing process, and make it a daily routine that you can enjoy together.

Remember to consult with a healthcare professional before incorporating juicing into your daily routine, especially if you have any underlying health conditions or are taking any medications.

With the right approach, juicing can be a beneficial addition to your daily routine for maximum health benefits.

CHAPTER VIII. JUICING FOR CANCER SURVIVORS

– Nutritional Needs During Recovery

Juicing has gained popularity among cancer survivors as a way to help meet their nutritional needs during recovery. Chemotherapy and radiation can often have harsh effects on the body, causing nausea, loss of appetite and trouble eating solid foods. Juicing can provide a concentrated dose of essential vitamins, minerals, and antioxidants that are important for supporting the healing process and boosting the immune system.

One of the most significant benefits of juicing for cancer survivors is the ability to easily consume large quantities of fruits and vegetables.

Juicing allows for the removal of insoluble fiber, which can be difficult for some cancer survivors to digest.

This makes the nutrients in these plants more easily available for absorption and use by the body.

When juicing for cancer recovery, it is essential to select fruits and vegetables that are rich in nutrients and antioxidants.

These include dark leafy greens, berries, cruciferous vegetables like broccoli and cauliflower, and citrus fruits. These nutrient-dense foods can help to support the body's natural defense mechanisms and fight off the damaging effects of treatments.

In addition to providing essential nutrients, juicing can also help to hydrate the body.

Staying well hydrated is crucial for cancer survivors to maintain their energy levels and replace fluids lost from treatment side effects.

– Juicing Recipes for Detoxification and Healing

Juicing has been gaining popularity in recent years as a natural way to detoxify the body and promote healing. It involves extracting the juice from fruits and vegetables, providing a concentrated source of vitamins, minerals, and phytonutrients that are essential for our overall health.

While juicing has countless benefits for everyone, it has been found to be particularly beneficial for cancer patients.

A study published in the Journal of Clinical Oncology found that cancer patients who incorporated fresh vegetable and fruit juices into their diet had significantly lower levels of toxic chemicals in their bodies compared to those who did not juice.

This is because the natural enzymes and antioxidants found in fresh juices help to break down and eliminate toxins in the body.

In addition, juicing provides a quick and easy way to consume a large amount of nutrients in one sitting, which is crucial for cancer patients who often have limited appetites.

There are many different types of juicing recipes for detoxification and healing, but for cancer patients, it is important to focus on recipes that are specifically tailored to support the body's immune system and promote healing.

The following are some key ingredients to include in juicing recipes for cancer patients:

1. Dark Leafy Greens: Leafy greens such as kale, spinach, and collard greens are rich in chlorophyll, a powerful detoxifying agent. They also contain antioxidants and essential vitamins and minerals that support the immune system.

2. Cruciferous Vegetables: Cruciferous vegetables like broccoli, cabbage, and cauliflower are known for their powerful anti-cancer properties.

They are rich in phytochemicals and sulfur compounds that help to fight cancer cells and detoxify the body.

3. Berries: Berries like blueberries, raspberries, and strawberries are packed with antioxidants that help to reduce inflammation and protect cells from damage caused by free radicals.

4. Turmeric: This yellow spice has been used for its healing properties for centuries. It contains a compound called curcumin which has powerful anti-inflammatory and anti-cancer effects.

5. Ginger: Ginger is another spice that has been used for its medicinal properties. It contains gingerol, which has been found to have anti-cancer properties and can also help to reduce nausea and inflammation.

Here are two easy and delicious juicing recipes that you can try at home for detoxification and healing:

1. Green Detox Juice:

- 1 cup kale

- 1 cup spinach

- 1 cucumber

- 1 green apple

- 1 lemon

- 1 inch of fresh ginger

Wash and chop all the ingredients and run them through a juicer. Drink immediately and enjoy the powerful detoxifying effects of this green juice.

2. Berry Blast Juice:

- 1 cup mixed berries (blueberries, raspberries, strawberries)

- 1 cucumber

- 1 medium-sized beetroot

- 1 lemon

- 1 inch of fresh turmeric

Wash and chop all the ingredients and juice them together. This delicious juice is full of antioxidants and anti-inflammatory properties that can help to boost the immune system and fight cancer cells.

In conclusion, juicing is an excellent way for cancer patients to support their bodies' natural detoxification processes and promote healing.

By incorporating specific ingredients into their juicing recipes, cancer patients can take advantage of the powerful healing properties of fruits, vegetables, and spices to aid in their recovery. Always consult with your doctor before making any changes to your diet, and be sure to use organic produce when possible for the best results.

– Boosting Immunity and Reducing Risk of Recurrence

Cancer patients face a long and challenging journey, not only through the treatment process but also in maintaining a healthy lifestyle.

After going through intense treatments that can weaken the immune system, it is crucial for cancer patients to focus on boosting their immune system and reducing the risk of recurrence.

Juicing is a great way to achieve these goals as it provides a high concentration of essential nutrients in a liquid form that is easy to digest and absorb.

Here are some key ingredients to include in juicing recipes for boosting immunity and reducing the risk of recurrence:

1. Citrus Fruits: Citrus fruits are packed with vitamin C, which is essential for boosting the immune system. They also contain bioflavonoids, which have been found to have anti-cancer properties.

2. Carrots: Carrots are rich in beta-carotene, which can help to enhance immune function and prevent cancer cell growth.

3. Garlic: Garlic is a powerful immune-booster that also has antioxidant and anti-inflammatory properties. It contains allicin, a compound that can help to reduce the risk of cancer recurrence.

4. Leafy Greens: Leafy greens are packed with essential vitamins and minerals, as well as antioxidants, that can help to strengthen the immune system and reduce inflammation.

5. Grapes: Grapes contain resveratrol, a compound that is known for its anti-cancer properties. It can also help to boost the immune system and reduce the risk of cancer recurrence.

Here are two delicious juicing recipes that can help to boost immunity and reduce the risk of recurrence:

1. Immune-Boosting Juice:

- 1 orange

- 1 grapefruit

- 2 carrots

- 1 inch of fresh ginger

- 1 small bunch of parsley

Juice all the ingredients together and enjoy the zesty and immune-boosting effects of this delicious juice.

2. Green Carrot Juice:

- 2 green apples

- 2 carrots

- 1 cucumber

- 1 cup spinach

- 1 cup kale

- 1 lemon

Run all the ingredients through a juicer and drink up for a high dose of immune-boosting nutrients and antioxidants.

In addition to incorporating these key ingredients into their juicing recipes, cancer patients should also focus on maintaining a healthy lifestyle by exercising regularly, getting enough rest, and managing stress.

It is also important to consult with a healthcare professional before making any changes to their diet.

In conclusion, juicing is a powerful tool for cancer patients looking to boost their immune system and reduce the risk of cancer recurrence.

By including specific ingredients in their juicing recipes and maintaining a healthy lifestyle, cancer patients can support their body's natural defense mechanisms and enhance their overall well-being.

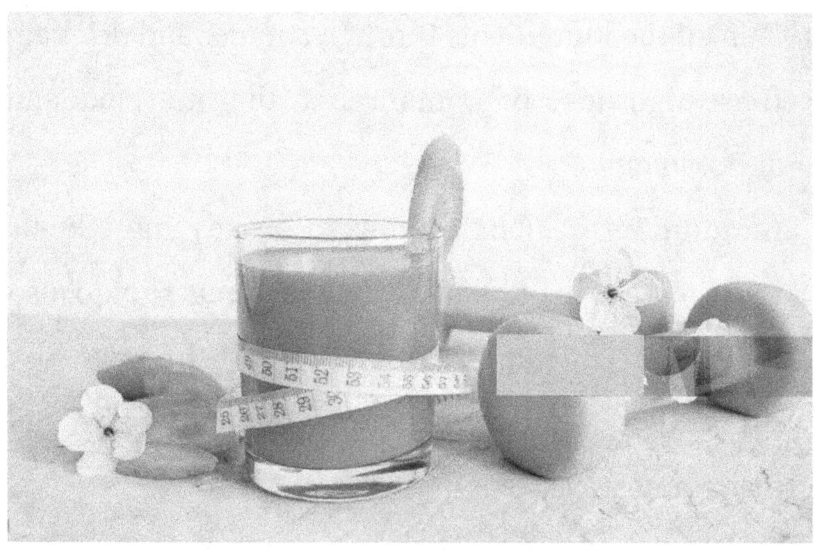

CHAPTER X. CONCLUSION

- Summary of Key Points

- Juicing is a natural and effective way to detoxify the body and promote healing.

- Incorporating fresh vegetable and fruit juices into the diet can lower levels of toxic chemicals in cancer patients' bodies.

- Key ingredients in juicing recipes for cancer patients include dark leafy greens, cruciferous vegetables, berries, turmeric, and ginger.

- Juicing can help boost immunity and reduce the risk of cancer recurrence.

- Recommended reading and resources include books like "The Juicing Bible" and "The Cancer-Fighting Kitchen" as well as organizations like the American Cancer Society and Cancer Care.

- Encouragement for Incorporating Juicing into a Cancer Journey

Dealing with a cancer diagnosis and treatment can be overwhelming, both physically and emotionally. It is natural to feel tired, fatigued, and lack appetite during this time. However, incorporating juicing into your cancer journey can provide numerous benefits for your health and well-being.

Firstly, juicing provides a concentrated source of essential nutrients, vitamins, and minerals that are easily absorbed by the body. This is important for cancer patients who often have a reduced appetite due to treatment.

Juicing can ensure that your body is getting the necessary nutrients to support and strengthen your immune system.

Moreover, juicing has been found to be particularly beneficial for cancer patients as it helps to eliminate toxins from the body.

Cancer patients often have high levels of toxic chemicals in their bodies due to treatment, which can lead to various health issues. By incorporating fresh juices into your diet, you can help to detoxify your body and promote healing.

In addition to the physical benefits, juicing can also provide emotional and mental support during your cancer journey.

Preparing and drinking fresh juices can be a calming and meditative experience, helping to reduce stress and anxiety. The act of nourishing your body with healthy and nutritious juices can also give a sense of control and empowerment during a time when many aspects of life may seem out of your control.

It is important to remember to consult with your healthcare provider before making any changes to your diet, especially if you are going through treatment.

They can provide personalized recommendations and guidelines for incorporating juicing into your cancer journey safely.

In conclusion, incorporating juicing into your cancer journey can provide numerous benefits for your physical, emotional, and mental well-being.

It can help to boost your immune system, detoxify your body, and provide a sense of control and empowerment during a challenging time.

With the right ingredients and guidance, juicing can be a simple and enjoyable way to support your body's healing process.

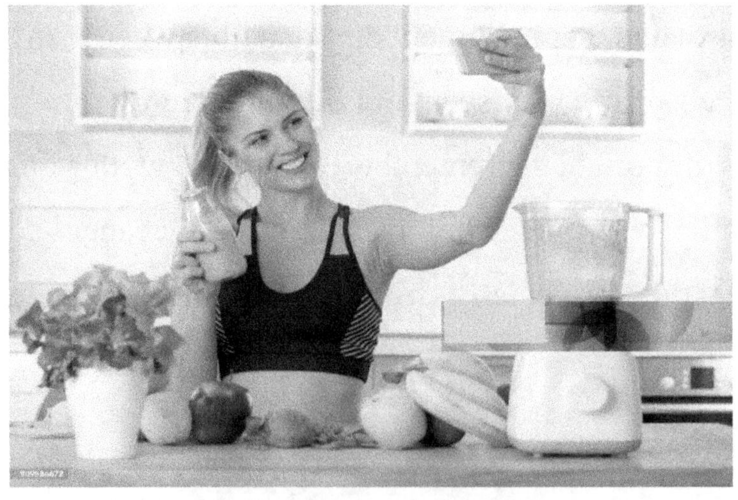

CHAPTER XI. INDEX OF RECIPES

- List of Juicing Recipes by Symptom and Type of Cancer

1. For Digestive Issues (stomach, colon, and esophageal cancers):

- Carrot and Ginger Juice: 2 carrots, 1 inch of fresh ginger

- Cabbage and Pineapple Juice: 1 cup cabbage, 1 cup pineapple

- Celery and Apple Juice: 2 stalks celery, 1 green apple

2. For Nausea and Chemotherapy Side Effects:

- Strawberry and Coconut Water Juice: 1 cup strawberries, 1 cup coconut water

- Lemon and Mint Juice: 1 lemon, handful of mint leaves, 1 cucumber

- Carrot and Orange Juice: 2 carrots, 1 orange

3. For Weak Immune System:

- Kale and Pineapple Juice: 1 cup kale, 1 cup pineapple

- Beetroot and Ginger Juice: 1 small beetroot, 1 inch of fresh ginger

- Spinach and Kiwi Juice: 1 cup spinach, 2 kiwis

4. For Lung Cancer:

- Blueberry and Spinach Juice: 1 cup blueberries, 1 cup spinach

- Grapefruit and Carrot Juice: 1 grapefruit, 2 carrots

- Cucumber and Celery Juice: 1 cucumber, 2 stalks celery

5. For Breast Cancer:

- Turmeric and Ginger Juice: 1 inch of fresh turmeric, 1 inch of fresh ginger

- Broccoli and Apple Juice: 1 cup broccoli, 1 green apple

- Pomegranate and Beetroot Juice: 1 small pomegranate, 1 small beetroot

6. For Prostate Cancer:

- Tomato and Basil Juice: 2 tomatoes, handful of basil leaves

- Watermelon and Spinach Juice: 1 cup watermelon, 1 cup spinach

- Carrot and Garlic Juice: 2 carrots, 2 cloves of garlic

7. For Skin Cancer:

- Green Tea and Lemon Juice: 1 cup green tea, 1 lemon

- Cucumber and Aloe Vera Juice: 1 cucumber, 1 small piece of aloe vera

- Orange and Carrot Juice: 1 orange, 2 carrots

Remember to consult with your doctor before incorporating any new ingredients into your diet, especially if you are undergoing cancer treatment. Be sure to use organic produce when possible for the best results.